CW00447615

More praise for
An Introduction to Chinese Medicine

Finally, a concise and approachable guide to Traditional Chinese Medicine! This is the type of resource I have wanted to share with my patients during my more than 40 years of clinical practice.

– Angela C. Wu, OMD, LAc
   Author of *Fertility Wisdom: How Traditional Chinese Medicine Can Help Overcome Infertility*

Toby Daly's new book fills a needed void for patients who desire to understand the basic foundations of Chinese Medicine. This is the first book I know of that breaks down the complexities of Chinese medicine into simple and accessible language. It covers the roots and branches of Chinese Medicine from acupuncture, herbal medicine, diet therapy, qi gong, tai chi, cupping and more. It addresses questions about research and evidence of efficacy. I will be recommending this book to my patients and keeping a copy in the waiting area.

– George Mandler, CNS, LDN, LicAc, FABORM

Toby Daly has written a comprehensive and insightful guide to Chinese medicine that is both informative and engaging. Whether you're a practitioner or a patient, this book is an invaluable resource that will help you unlock the secrets of this ancient healing art.

– Lorne Brown, B.Sc., Dr.TCM, CPA CHt
   Founder of Healthy Seminars & Clinical Director of Acubalance Wellness Centre

Dr. Toby Daly has diligently shared his teacher's guidance for decades. In this book he continues to communicate the power and profundity of Chinese medicine in clear, precise and understandable language, to help you find the way to live a simple and happy life with a flexible mind and body. There is no greater guidance.

– Brandt Stickley, LAc
   Associate Professor, College of Classical Chinese Medicine

As a clinical practitioner of Chinese Medicine, my job involves more than the diagnosis and treatment of disease. I practice a medicine developed in a different time and place, and that often seems mysterious to the patients who come to see me, often because other, more conventional approaches have not yielded the results they seek. Often, these patients have an innate curiosity about what I'm doing. Why do I ask the questions I ask? Why do I palpate their wrists or abdomens? Why do I look at their tongues? And finally, how do I make sense of the seemingly disparate bits of information I glean from these different approaches?

Toby Daly has rendered us a great service, in that he has published a book which summarizes much of what we are called to communicate on a regular basis. The book is simple without being simplistic, and clearly explains what Chinese Medicine is, how it can be used, how it differs from other medical models, what evidence base backs it use, and more.

There are a small number of books I am happy to recommend to those patients who are curious about delving deeper into Chinese Medicine, and Toby's book will now be at the top of my list as a general primer and introduction into this beautiful medicine.

– Phil Settels, LAc, DAOM
    Dean of Academic Affairs, DAOM Program
    Academy of Chinese Culture and Health Sciences

An Introduction to Chinese Medicine is straightforward but not oversimplified, descriptive but not mystifying, detailed but not tedious. Toby Daly answers the questions his new patients have asked in a thorough yet easy-to-understand manner. This book gives an overview of the various treatment methods found in the clinic and explains them based on both clinical research and Chinese medical theory without compromising either side. This is the book you should read before your first treatment.

– Lorraine Wilcox, PhD, LAc
    Author of *Moxibustion: A Modern Clinical Handbook*

Editor: Daniel Maxwell
Cover design: Jennifer Black
Page layout: Daniel Meagher

An Introduction to Chinese Medicine: A Patient's Guide to Acupuncture, Herbal Medicine, Nutrition & More

To Laurie, for your boundless love and sincerity

Contents

Acknowledgements

I am forever indebted to my teacher, the wandering monk, who set me upon the path of medicine, to Dr. Angela C. Wu who mentored me in the art of clinical practice, and to Jeffery Yuen who taught me how to peer through the many lenses of Chinese medicine. I am appreciative of the scholars listed in the references section who provided material throughout this book.

To the patients with questions about Chinese medicine, especially the patients not satisfied with my initial answers but pressed me for deeper answers, your curiosity planted the seeds for this text. This book is immeasurably better due to Daniel 'The Free and Easy Editor' Maxwell's guidance. Thank you especially to Lorne Brown, Ted Chen, Edward Chiu, Julian Cohen, John and Janet Daly, Peter Deadman, Heiner Fruehauf, Stephanie Hoover, Noel Kosiek, George Mandler, Michael Max, Linda Reed, Phil Settels, Brandt Stickley, Sharon Weizenbaum, and Lorraine Wilcox.

Foreword

How best to explain Chinese medicine to people who do not know about it? Should we dumb it down, presuming that concepts like qi and the acupuncture channels are labels given by the ancient Chinese to things they did not and could not understand, like oxygen and nerves? Or do we retreat to our jade towers, don our silk pajamas and pronounce from on high lofty judgements in a strange tongue to dazzle the credulous (and confound the skeptical)? Today we see a plethora of approaches to communicating Chinese medicine; professional websites, social media and clinical research papers all have their own take, in which Chinese medicine is usually made to serve the ends of the person describing it. In this multiverse of perspectives, Chinese medicine can on the one hand occur as Orientalist hippy eco-medicine, or can be glossed in ultra-traditional classical rigour, or else be presented as a cutting-edge systems biological therapy. Such polarisations tend to be unsatisfactorily limiting, however, and do Chinese medicine - and the patients who could benefit from it - a disservice.

To communicate Chinese medicine successfully to the general public is a delicate business. It would require an author with a deep and broad understanding of the medicine. Someone who has been diligent with their study, and lucky with their teachers. Someone who is smart - but mentally flexible enough - to transmit knowledge without dumbing it down nor retreating into abstruseness. A light touch would be needed, along with a sharp mind in order to cut out everything that does not need to be said. Humour and humility would also be useful to hold the paradox of this medicine, which encompasses both the infinite complexity of human illness as well as its elegant, ordered simplicity when rendered into yin-yang terms.

Look no further. That author, that book, are here. Toby Daly has produced a text that is a service not just for prospective or existing patients of Chinese medicine, but for practitioners too. As a practitioner, I have lost count of the number of times I have been asked by patients for 'further reading' on Chinese medicine,

13

and I am frequently at a loss where to direct them. The public-facing information available is limited in the ways described above, while the books I feel I can authentically recommend tend to be practitioner level texts. No longer. In my mind's eye I see small stacks of this book in Chinese medicine clinic reception areas, with copies being perused by curious patients. Practitioners will also be able to direct interested patients to buy a copy online. In this way authentic, solid information about this medicine can be disseminated to those who need to know.

And let's face it, more people need to know. Read on…

Daniel Maxwell
Bath, England, March 2023

Prologue

I started as a patient myself.

Twenty-five years ago, I moved into a houseboat on Dal Lake in the Northern Indian state of Kashmir. I was seven months into a trip that was originally supposed to last two months but would ultimately span two years. In the neighboring houseboat was a wandering Korean Buddhist monk. Even though we were from completely different backgrounds, I felt an immediate and deep kinship with him.

Travelling on a budget in India had wreaked havoc on my digestive system. I had been plagued with diarrhea for months and had completely lost my appetite. My normal weight of 190 pounds on a six-foot four-inch frame had been reduced to a mere 150 pounds.

The monk and I travelled together for the next six weeks from Kashmir to Ladakh and on into Himachal Pradesh. It was apparent from my frequent trips to the bathroom and emaciated body how ill I was. My new travelling companion repeatedly offered to help me with his acupuncture needles. Since my grandfather had been a medical doctor, and my background was in science, I was reluctant. I felt very confident that needles without any medicine going through them intravenously could do nothing for me. After a few weeks of travelling, I relented, thinking, 'He's such a nice man, this won't do anything for me, but it will make him feel better if he thinks he's helping me.'

He inserted four needles into my hands and feet, and I rested for twenty minutes. I got up from my first acupuncture treatment and ate an entire meal with three desserts. I could not believe it. My digestive system normalized and my fascination for and appreciation of acupuncture was born.

Before this first acupuncture treatment I had not merely been skeptical of Chinese medicine - I had been downright hostile towards it. I did not know any better. In the following chapters I will share what I have learned about Chinese medicine since that initial encounter twenty-five years ago. Here you will find the answers I have given to common questions from thousands of patients during my last two decades of work as a practitioner of Chinese medicine.

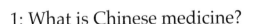

1: What is Chinese medicine?

Chinese medicine is like an ocean made up of many different currents. These currents include acupuncture, moxibustion, herbal formulas, cupping, manual therapies, nutritional strategies, exercises, lifestyle modifications, and many others. These currents have ebbed and flowed in popularity throughout the centuries. What they all have in common is a core framework based on the theory of yin and yang.

Yin 陰 and yang 陽 (pronounced 'yahng') are the two fundamental categories in Chinese medicine through which everything in the universe can be understood. Light and dark, hot and cold, dry and wet, inside and outside…everything can be seen in terms of yin and yang. For Chinese medicine practitioners, health in the human body is simply yin and yang in a state of dynamic balance. Illness occurs when this balance is disturbed. The goal of Chinese medicine, regardless of the modality, is to restore this equilibrium.

When I look through the yin-yang lens and observe a patient with a high fever, I am likely to diagnose the patient as having too much yang and not enough yin. I could use acupuncture points, an herbal formula, dietary recommendations, or any other modality in Chinese medicine to reduce yang and supplement yin. An overweight, cold, and tired patient with too much yin and not enough yang would require, regardless of modality, the opposite strategy.

Chinese physicians have been peering through the yin-yang lens to help their patients since at least the publication of the *Huang Di Nei Jing* (Yellow Emperor's Inner Classic) in the second century BCE. Since then, countless authors have shared their successful strategies for balancing yin and yang to counteract epidemics, overcome infertility, set broken bones, restore digestive systems, heal dermatological conditions, alleviate sciatica, and address the endless other ways the human body can become ill.

Unlike Europe, China never experienced a dark age, so these medical ideas have been continuously studied, applied, and refined with each generation. Today, we are fortunate to be able to access a medical system that has been clinically tested and verified for millennia. Century after century, it has developed new strategies and discarded ineffective or harmful approaches. Because of this careful curation, modern practitioners have inherited a trove of safe and effective approaches to alleviate disease.

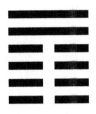

2: How does Chinese medicine diagnose an illness?

A Chinese medicine diagnosis is formed from the medical interview, observation, and palpation.

Patients new to Chinese medicine are often surprised when they see a clinician - for, say, low back pain - and are asked questions about their diet, sleep, and sweating patterns. To effectively address the back pain, the Chinese medicine clinician must understand 'who' has the back pain. The back pain does not exist in a space separate from the rest of the person - it is embedded within the matrix of their entire body and mind.

The more deeply a clinician can understand the individual who has the back pain, the more completely they can identify what is enabling the back pain to present in the body. For example, a clinician will make an entirely different diagnosis for a patient with low back pain who sweats normally versus a patient with back pain who experiences drenching night sweats. By considering the individual as a whole, the fundamental cause of the back pain can be identified. Only then can it be cured, rather than just covered up or temporarily improved.

Since there were no blood tests, MRI, or PET scans when Chinese medicine was being developed in the Han dynasty (206 BCE - 220 CE), physicians had to rely not only on asking questions, but also observation and palpation of the surface of the body, to determine the pathology underneath. There are many diagnostic systems in

Chinese medicine, but the most common involve assessing the patient's tongue, pulse, and abdomen.

When a Chinese medicine clinician observes your tongue, they are looking at the color and shape of the tongue body, the quality and texture of the tongue coating, and the presentation of the veins under the tongue. The clinician correlates these findings to a yin and yang diagnostic framework. For example, a deep red tongue likely indicates the body is too yang and a pale tongue indicates the body is too yin.

Patients are sometimes surprised when a Chinese medicine physician palpates the arteries on both of their wrists. The practitioner, however, is not only interested in the patient's heart rate. Chinese medicine has a sophisticated and comprehensive system that correlates palpable qualities found at different sections and depths of the radial artery with the relative strength of yin and yang in the body.

There is a saying in Chinese medicine: 'As above, so below.' Many methods of abdominal palpation work on this principle. Discomfort elicited on palpation directly above an organ or along an acupuncture channel tend to indicate pathology in that organ or channel. There are also areas on the abdomen that do not correspond to the organs directly beneath the area but reflect other parts of the body. For example, the acupuncture tradition I practice assesses the state of the liver, which is anatomically located on the right side of the abdomen, by palpating the left side of the abdomen, just below the ribs.

A clinician gathers all their findings from the medical interview, careful observation, and methodical palpation, and then distills them to formulate a diagnostic pattern. The diagnostic pattern is a dynamic blueprint showing the relative excess or deficiency of yin and yang in the patient - and therefore how to address their imbalance. For example, a patient at my clinic recently complained of debilitating hot flashes. She described them as a tidal wave of heat permeating her entire body. When a hot flash surged, her clothes felt smothering and constricting. I noticed that she had a red flushed face. Palpating her radial arteries, I found her pulses were rapid and strong.

Together, these findings revealed her diagnostic pattern to be one of yang excess. I used the modalities that will be discussed in later chapters - acupuncture, herbal medicine, and dietary recommendations - to address her yang excess. Another recent patient presented with a chronic cough, chills, a pale tongue, pallid complexion, and slow pulses that felt tight like a bowstring. He felt utterly exhausted. To successfully alleviate his cough, chills, and exhaustion I needed to counterbalance his pattern of yin excess by supplementing yang. To do this, I employed the appropriate acupuncture, moxibustion, herbal medicine and lifestyle modifications specific for his presentation.

Both patients had their symptoms resolved, but not by suppressing their symptoms with exogenous hormones or Dextromethorphan. They were resolved by restoring the dynamic balance of yin and yang. The first patient's symptoms were manifesting due to the disharmony created by an excess of yang and a relative deficiency of yin. The second patient had the exact opposite presentation, an excess of yin and a relative deficiency of yang. For both patients, treatment reset the yin-yang balance, and the hot flashes and chronic cough were no longer able to manifest in their bodies.

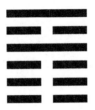

3: Is Chinese medicine an alternative medicine?

Is Chinese food an alternative food? Is Chinese language an alternative language?

Chinese medicine is simply the collection of successful healing strategies gathered as Chinese civilization endured over the last two millennia. Because it did not develop in Europe or India, it is based on the innate cultural ideas and language of China - yin and yang - rather than the 'cell theory' of modern biomedicine or the 'doshas and prana' paradigm of traditional Indian medicine.

Because Chinese language and ideas are fundamentally different from the language and ideas of Europe or America, they can feel unfamiliar - and therefore uncomfortable. This discomfort can threaten to derail our fruitful engagement with Chinese medicine. However, any medical system should be judged not on how closely it matches our familiar cultural references, but solely on its clinical effectiveness and safety.

No matter which medical system is used to observe it, the human body is the same. Each medical system - whether Chinese, biomedicine or Ayurvedic - has inherent strengths and weaknesses. As we will see in the following sections, although Chinese medicine is not the optimal choice for every ailment, it occupies a uniquely safe and effective niche in the medical systems currently available to patients. It is not therefore an alternative medicine, but like Chinese language and Chinese food, it is simply medicine developed in China.

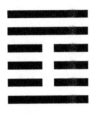

4: What is acupuncture? How does it work? Does it hurt?

The word 'acupuncture' is derived from the Latin term 'acupunctura' meaning 'puncturing with sharp objects'. It was coined when British and American doctors visiting China first encountered a modality they had never seen before - the insertion of thin needles into a body to elicit a therapeutic effect. Every human body has acupuncture points and channels, but only the Chinese discovered, mapped, and exploited this feature of our shared biology.

The Chinese term for acupuncture is zhen 針 (meaning needle) and it is often paired with the character jiu 灸 (referring to moxibustion, the topic for our next chapter). How the Chinese first started to utilize acupuncture to treat disease is unknown. The first time that a sophisticated system of theory and acupuncture practice was presented was in the *Huang Di Nei Jing* in the second century BCE. Since then, countless texts and oral traditions have emerged that inform the myriad styles of acupuncture seen today.

These styles range from orthopedic approaches that focus on the treatment of musculoskeletal problems, to styles that consider the whole mental and physical complex of the patient, including seasonal and climatic - and in some cases even astronomical - influences on health. Simplistic modern approaches to acupuncture such as 'dry needling' have more recently been developed; these are often taught in a weekend as an extra tool for physical therapists or osteopaths.

However, this stripped-down over-simplified approach can be problematic, not only because it lacks the historical knowledge base referred to above, but also because the training usually involves insufficient hours to make the practitioner safe and effective. As acupuncturist Benjamin Hawes notes - 'Our needles have always been dry'. Of the traditional East Asian approaches, although on the surface the different styles may appear unique, they are all still rooted in the fundamental theory of yin and yang.

Hundreds of research studies have confirmed the effectiveness of acupuncture (see Chapter 13 and Appendix A) but the exact mechanism of its effects is not yet fully understood by science. Brain imaging studies have shown that acupuncture affects nervous system function. Acupuncture needles have also been shown to affect the fascia, the connective tissue that surrounds and connects every structure in the human body. Grooves in the fascia corresponding to acupuncture channels may be the pathways that allow acupuncture needles to have wide-ranging effects on parts of the body far away from the location of the needle, including the internal organs. It is theorized that this combination of effects from acupuncture needles on the nervous system and fascia yields the systemic therapeutic changes that result from acupuncture treatment.

Almost every patient considering acupuncture wants to know, 'Does it hurt?'. The answer depends on the patient's level of sensitivity and the part of the body into which the acupuncture needle is being inserted. There are acupuncture points across the entire body. In general points on the torso are minimally painful or not painful at all. Points on the head, arms, and legs tend to be more sensitive - especially points on the hands and feet. Fortunately, acupuncture needles are nothing like hypodermic needles, which are designed to penetrate blood vessels and tissue; acupuncture needles in comparison are extremely fine, and when inserted tend to glide past physical structures like blood vessels and nerves under the skin.

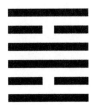

5: What is moxibustion?

The earliest text reference for what we now refer to as the acupuncture channels is the *Wu Shi Er Bing Fang* (Prescriptions for Fifty-Two Diseases). This text was written on silk in the Western Han dynasty (206 BCE – 9 CE) and was unearthed from a tomb in the 1970s. It describes the channels associated with acupuncture, although rather than acupuncture needles this text recommends using moxibustion on the channels to achieve a therapeutic effect.

The word 'moxibustion' is derived by combining the Japanese word for 'burning' (mokusa) with the Latin word for 'burning' (combustum). Moxibustion involves burning dried mugwort leaves (Artemisiae argyi Folium) on or near acupuncture points and channels. There are many ways practitioners of Chinese medicine use moxibustion to conduct therapeutic heat into the body. Some traditions use tiny rice grain-sized cones of moxa directly on the acupuncture points. Other traditions use cigar-shaped rolls of mugwort, or a box in which the burning mugwort can be suspended over areas of the patient's body.

Moxibustion is mostly used for patients with a diagnosis of yang deficiency or yin excess. The therapeutic heat from the ignited mugwort gently supplements yang. I frequently counterbalance the damp, cold, and dark yin season of winter with the dry, warm, and bright yang of moxibustion. Patients enjoy the smokey but pleasant experience of this modality.

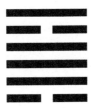

6: What is Chinese herbal medicine? (Why are you giving me these mushrooms, roots, twigs, and berries?)

Humans have been using plant, animal, and mineral substances as medicine for millennia. One of the earliest known archeological sites confirming this has been dated back 60,000 years.[1] A substance discovered at this ancient site is a common herb in the Chinese materia medica – Ma Huang (Ephedrae Herba).

The oldest Chinese compendium of medicinal substances that has survived until the present day is the *Shen Nong Ben Cao Jing* (Divine Farmer's Classic of Materia Medica). It was compiled in the Eastern Han dynasty, almost 2,000 years ago. This text contains 365 entries, each describing the medicinal qualities of a substance, how it should be used, and the duration of its use.

There have been countless oral and written herbal traditions in the centuries since then. Any traditions that have survived until the present day have been collected in an official materia medica, the *Zhong Yao Da Ci Dian* (Encyclopedia of Chinese Materia Medica), which contains more than five thousand entries. Modern practitioners can prescribe any of these substances, but only around five hundred are commonly used.

Each substance in the Chinese materia medica is categorized according to its yin and yang qualities. These qualities are determined by the substance's flavor and temperature, as well as other aspects such as density, weight, and appearance.

A substance may be light (yang) like a leaf or flower, or heavy (yin) like a root or mineral. Flavors such as sweet and spicy are yang, while bitter and salty are yin. Warm or hot temperatures are yang. Cool or cold temperatures are yin. A substance with a supplementing action is yang, while one with a draining actions is yin.

As an example, the famous Chinese medicinal ginseng ('Ren Shen' in Chinese) is classified as sweet (yang), slightly bitter (yin), and warm (yang). Its main actions are to supplement (yang) the heart, lung, and digestive systems, generate fluids (yin), and calm the mind (yin). Ginseng's unique combination of yin and yang qualities makes it suitable to address a pattern of deficiency (yin) presenting with symptoms like shortness of breath, fatigue, poor appetite, palpitations with anxiety, insomnia, and poor memory.

In Chinese medicine clinical practice herbs are rarely prescribed individually but rather combined into formulas to enhance their beneficial properties and mitigate any side effects that might be caused by individual herbs. Chinese medicine clinicians still routinely prescribe the 113 herbal formulas compiled in the 1,800-year-old text, the *Shang Han Lun* (Discussion on Cold Damage).

Or clinicians can turn to the *Bei Ji Qian Yin Yao Fang* (Prescriptions Worth a Thousand in Gold for Every Emergency), a Tang dynasty text which contains 5,300 entries. Modern clinicians can now source their prescriptions from a database of formulas maintained by the Chinese Academy of Traditional Chinese Medicine, which contains 85,989 ancient and modern formulas.

Once a formula is selected it needs to be prepared. Modern Chinese herbal medicine is delivered in three main ways - decoctions, tinctures, and granules. Decoctions are made by boiling herbs in water, often twice, to extract their active ingredients for ingestion. Tinctures are made by using the solvent, preservative, and yang qualities of alcohol to extract the bioactive ingredients of the herbs.

Granules are the most modern delivery system. They are prepared by binding the concentrated liquid of decocted herbs to excipients (usually starch or the raw herb itself). Granules are then either dispensed loose, in which case the patient merely adds hot water to reconstitute the formula, or they are packed into gelatin or cellulose capsules for easy ingestion.

I use all three of these formula preparation methods in my clinic and I am grateful for the flexibility they provide. Some patients love to see the individual raw herbs as they are dispensed, and then enjoy the aromatic scents produced as they are cooked. For these formulas I source locally grown herbs where possible and I can easily add or remove individual herbs from a formula. Some patients are too busy to cook a formula, or they prefer their kitchen to not smell like a Song dynasty apothecary. These patients appreciate the convenience of tinctures and granules. Whatever the delivery method, patients receive the benefits of centuries of clinical insight and the safety inherent in formulas that literally hundreds of millions of patients have taken for more than a millennium.

[1] Solecki, R.S. (1955). Shanidar cave, a paleolithic site in northern Iraq, *Annual Report of the Board of Regents of the Smithsonian Institution*, 389–425.

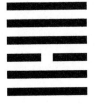

7: What is cupping?

You may have seen circular discolorations on the back of athletes such as twenty-three Olympic gold medal winner Michael Phelps, or on the shoulders of four-time NBA champion Stephen Curry. These marks are from cupping. This Chinese medical modality uses a vacuum created in small glass or plastic cups that suck onto the skin. Historically, the first cups were made from a section of bamboo with one hollow end.

A cupping treatment may consist of a single cup, or multiple cups may be used all at once. The cups may be placed on specific acupuncture points and/or muscle groups, or the practitioner may slide them along the acupuncture channels. They are usually retained on the skin for five to fifteen minutes. The vacuum is made either through introducing a flame into the cup, or by using a small pump. If 'fire cupping' is used (with a flame creating the vacuum), the treatment will be especially helpful to address yin excess conditions such as pain that is worse with cold weather.

The goal of cupping is to improve circulation, promote healing, and alleviate pain. Cupping achieves this by expanding the capillaries (the fine branching blood vessels in the body) to increase the amount of fluid moving through the muscle tissue. Cupping can also speed up lymphatic circulation.

Cupping can be used to address acute and chronic injuries, acute and chronic inflammation, and is useful for dermatological conditions. It has been safely and effectively used in Chinese medicine for centuries. Like many aspects of Chinese medicine, the mechanism for the effectiveness of cupping has not been properly studied and understood, although a small systematic review in 2011 showed cupping therapy significantly reduced low back pain and pain associated with cancer.[1]

I have cupped thousands of patients, and cupping along with moxibustion are some of my patient's favorite modalities. The gentle negative pressure sensation of cupping is profoundly relaxing, and patients liken it to getting a deep tissue massage. A few friendships have even been kindled when fellow patients have spotted cupping marks at the pool or gym!

[1] Kim J.I., Lee, M.S., Lee, D.H. et al. (2011). Cupping for Treating Pain: A Systemic Review, *Evidence-Based Complementary and Alternative Medicine*, DOI:10.1093/ecam/nep035.

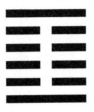

8: How does Chinese medicine use diet to prevent and treat disease?

There is a blurry line dividing herbal medicine and food in Chinese medicine. Ginger, for example, is a Chinese culinary staple that is also found in many of the most powerful Chinese medicinal formulas.

In Western nutrition, dietary strategies are often based on scientific theory regarding macronutrient ratios (carbohydrate, protein, and fat), but do not tend to take account of an individual's unique constitution. Because of this generalization broad dietary guidelines tend to be recommended to the whole population, and we see trends like 'Everyone should eat low fat foods' and lately 'Everyone should eat low carbohydrate foods'. Since protein is the only remaining macronutrient without a fad diet, it is only a matter of time until we see 'Everyone should eat low protein foods'.

Western nutrition is a relatively new discipline without deep roots. Because of this its recommendations swing wildly as each new research study contradicts the previous one. This results in headlines such as 'The Ten Health Benefits of Drinking Red Wine' and the following week 'Ugly Side Effects of Wine You Don't Even Know About, According to Science'.

In Chinese medical nutrition every person and each individual food is understood to have a unique combination of yin and yang qualities. When I have a patient with excess yang in their body, for example someone that is thirsty and restless with dry skin and scant urination, I will advise them to emphasize yin natured foods in their diet to restore balance, like apple, avocado, barley, broccoli, cabbage, cantaloupe, green tea, mulberry, pear, peppermint, pumpkin, radish, spinach, strawberry, tofu, yogurt, and zucchini.

For a patient with excess yin in their body (for example someone that gets chilled easily, has low energy, and edema), I will advise them to consume slightly yang natured foods like basil, beef, black pepper, cherry, chestnut, chicken, cinnamon, clove, garlic, lamb, leek, lentil, mustard greens, nutmeg, onion, peanut, sunflower seed, turmeric, venison, and walnut to restore their yang.

Although each individual food has its own yin and yang qualities, these are not immutable. Preparation methods can enhance or diminish these qualities. Cooking methods such as grilling and roasting increase the yang quality of food, while salt-frying and honey-frying - or omitting cooking entirely - increase the yin quality of foods.

While the focus of Chinese medical dietary strategies is on individually tailored prescription of specific foods to restore yin-yang balance, there are some near universal recommendations that are helpful for everyone. For example:

• Only eat until your stomach is 75 percent full; this will leave room for digestion
• Your biggest meal of the day should be at breakfast
• Minimize eating uncooked or cold food, especially in the winter
• Vegetables are more beneficial than fruit

I remind my patients that every meal we take into our bodies is an opportunity to enhance or degrade our health. Since Chinese medical nutrition considers the unique qualities of the individual as well as the unique qualities of each food, practitioners can use this sophisticated system to precisely answer the perennial question, 'What is a healthy diet?'

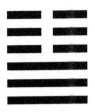

9: What are qi gong 氣功 and tai ji quan 太極拳?

Qi gong (pronounced 'chee gong') literally means 'working with your vitality', and is actually a relatively modern term, first coined in 1949. Since then, it has become an umbrella term for the meditative exercises that have been used to cultivate health and well-being in China for the last couple of millennia.

It is uncertain exactly how long qi gong has been practiced in China. One of the earliest clues we have is from the work of archeologists who recently recovered an engraved block of jade that clearly depicts a qi gong breathing technique. This jade relic was unearthed while excavating a tomb dated to the 4th century BCE.

The most well-known qi gong practice is tai ji quan (pronounced 'tai jee chuan'). Tai ji quan is often also written 't'ai chi chuan' or abbreviated to simply 'tai chi'. The Chinese language is logographic and different romanization systems can render the same Chinese characters, in this case 太極拳, differently into English. Whatever the romanization system used, the characters for tai ji quan translate to 'supreme ultimate boxing'. It is a martial art and a form of stylized meditative exercise that is commonly practiced outdoors in the morning in China, and recently more frequently in the West.

Qi gong methods can be used to supplement the yin and/or yang in the practitioner. In the same way that a physical therapist might prescribe a personalized exercise program based on their assessment of a patient's health, a practitioner of Chinese medicine can prescribe a personalized qi gong routine for their patient. The routine will be based on the patient's pattern diagnosis, and it will be prescribed specifically to balance this pattern.

I recommend qi gong practices to patients suffering from anxiety and stress, especially if these are due to a serious illness, like cancer. I recommend tai ji quan practice for my older patients who have difficulty with their balance. My personal experience with an assortment of qi gong practices, including tai ji quan, has been very rewarding. I have noticed increased equanimity and overall wellness, and at times even bliss.

There have been a handful of studies documenting the benefits of qi gong practices. We will discuss these and other Chinese medical research studies in Chapter 13.

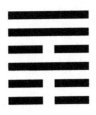

10: What is gua sha 刮痧?

Dr. Arya Nielsen describes gua sha as an 'instrument-assisted unidirectional press-stroking of a lubricated area of the body surface that intentionally creates transitory therapeutic petechiae representing extravasation of blood in the subcutis'.[1] Let us unpack this complete but technical statement:

'Instrument-assisted' refers to the tools used to perform gua sha. The material that these tools are made from vary widely, but they all have a smooth uniform edge. Historically, coins or porcelain spoons were used, or dedicated gua sha tools were made from jade, metal, or even animal horn. Practitioners today use disposable gua sha instruments that are used once and discarded, or instruments designed to be disinfected between uses.

'Unidirectional press-stroking' describes the rhythmic movement of the gua sha tool, which is used to stroke the skin repeatedly in one direction at a constant angle for six to fifteen strokes. The number of strokes is dependent on the amount of pressure applied by the practitioner and the response of the patient's skin to the therapy. A gua sha stroke is typically four to six inches long. All areas of the body where the skin is intact and not damaged are appropriate for gua sha, although it is most commonly applied to the neck and back.

'Lubricated area of the body surface' refers to the necessary application of a substance to reduce friction between the tool and the patient's skin. Peanut oil and black sesame seed oil are commonly used in China. Gua sha practitioners in the West commonly use olive oil alone or combined with other ingredients like beeswax or medicinal herbs.

'Transitory therapeutic petechiae' refers to the tiny red or purplish, raised dots that appear on the skin as an immediate response to a gua sha treatment. These raised dots quickly fade over a few days. 'Extravasation of blood in the subcutis' refers to the small amounts of blood that are freed from the tiny blood vessels just under the skin that result in the petechiae. This is not the same as bruising, which involves much more significant damage to the tissues.

Gua sha literally means 'scraping sand'. The 'scraping' refers to the unidirectional press-stroking and the 'sand' refers to the small petechiae that appear in response to the gua sha treatment. Gua sha stimulates the immune system, reduces pain, stops spasms, brings down inflammation, and can even help alleviate coughing and wheezing.

Patients report that the sensation of gua sha ranges from 'mostly comfortable' to 'slightly uncomfortable' during the treatment. The slight discomfort is especially likely as the practitioner nears the end of the treatment. My own experience as a patient with gua sha is of an experience that is thoroughly comfortable and deeply relaxing. The sensation - something like a deep itch being released from my muscles - was incredibly pleasant. However, remember to always communicate how you are feeling during the treatment with your gua sha practitioner so that they can make any adjustments.

[1] Nielsen, A. (2013). *Gua Sha: A Traditional Technique for Modern Practice.* Churchill Livingstone: Edinburgh.

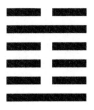

11: What is tui na 推拿?

The Chinese term for massage therapy is 'an mo', meaning 'pressing and rubbing'. Tui na, literally 'pushing and pulling', is the most frequently used form of massage therapy. An mo has a long history of continuous application in China, and we find the earliest text references for tui na begin in the Zhou Dynasty (700 - 481 BC).

There are many tui na techniques, but foundational ones are:

- **Rolling (gun fa)** – a smooth, rhythmic rolling movement of the practitioner's knuckles across the area to be treated
- **Acupressure (yi zhi chan tui fa)** – a focused and repetitive rocking motion with the practitioner's thumb on an acupuncture point
- **Pushing (tui fa)** – sliding pressure from the practitioner's whole hand, usually along an acupuncture channel
- **Kneading (rou fa)** – soft, repetitive and relatively slow circular strokes applied anywhere in the body
- **Pressing (an fa)** – relaxed pressure often using the practitioner's thumb or palm
- **Rubbing (mo fa)** – soothing circular pressure using the practitioner's palms and fingers
- **Grasping (na fa)** – one of the most frequently used tui na techniques: the practitioner uses their finger pads to squeeze and release large muscles

- **Finger striking (ji dian fa)** – the practitioner uses one finger or a grouping of their fingers to repeatedly strike an acupuncture point, a section of an acupuncture channel or a joint; ideally performed at two to three strikes per second
- **Chopping (ji fa)** – rhythmic strikes with the edge of the hand, usually on the patient's back; eliminates yin pathogens, like dampness, from the lungs and acupuncture channels
- **Vibrating (zhen fa)** – the practitioner uses their palm or finger to create a subtle quivering motion; the patient often experiences a sense of deep relaxation
- **Plucking (tan bo fa)** – the practitioner draws their thumb pad across muscles or tissues to release adhesions; especially helpful to address past traumatic injuries

There are yin and yang styles of tui na. The yin style uses a smaller range of these techniques, which are applied gently, slowly, and subtly to a treatment area. The yang style uses a larger range of more dynamic, vigorous techniques. In general, yin style tui na is more appropriate for chronic conditions and yang style tui na is more appropriate for acute pathologies.

I have received and performed both yin and yang style tui na. When I received yin style tui na, I felt deep relaxation as the practitioner gently loosened my tight muscles. Yang style tui na helped to release deep tension in my lower back. Tui na, especially yang style, can feel intense, so always communicate how you are feeling during the treatment. This will allow your tui na practitioner to make any necessary adjustments.

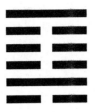

12: What is yang sheng 養生?

*The sages did not treat those already ill, but treated those
not yet ill, they did not put in order what was already
in disorder but put in order what was not yet in disorder.
When attempts at restoring order are initiated only after
disorder has fully developed, this is as if a well were dug
when one is thirsty, and as if weapons were cast when
the fight is on. Would this not be too late?*[1]

This passage is from the 2,200-year-old *Huang Di Nei Jing Su
Wen*; it illustrates the core preference in Chinese medicine for
seeking preventative measures rather than waiting for a disease to
manifest and grow in strength. This can be likened to how easy it
is to undo a small knot before it becomes too tight and tangled;
similarly Chinese medicine recommends intervening early using
gentle approaches.

This strategy of early intervention is much safer and more successful
than waiting until only more intense and therefore risky methods
are suitable for treatment. To accomplish this, Chinese medicine
has developed a wide range of behaviors, practices, and lifestyle
modifications, all gathered under the rubric of yang sheng.

Yang sheng means 'nourishing life' and encompasses strategies
to regulate mental and emotional states, ethical behavior, dietary
habits (including when and how we eat), exercise, sleep, healthy
sexual practices, and living in harmony with the changing seasonal
environment. All these strategies are aimed at preventing disease
and enhancing longevity.

Yang sheng methods are designed to supplement both the yin and yang qualities of our bodies and minds. Because our modern culture is strongly dominated by yang qualities - through ubiquitous bright shiny screens, artificial lighting throughout the night, 'heroic' work hours, minimal and fractured sleep, limited downtime, and noise day and night - yin methods are desperately needed to balance our lives.

We are even upsetting the yin and yang equilibrium of the entire planet by stripping 95 million barrels of oil from the earth every day. The natural state of crude oil is yin - underground, dark, liquid, and cool. By recasting it into a state of yang - above ground, bright, and hot - we are inviting global imbalance.

I often prescribe yang sheng practices to supplement patients' yin and counterbalance the prevailing yang of our modern restless culture. For the mind I recommend the quiet stillness of seated meditation. For physical exercise I suggest the slow graceful practice of tai ji quan or long slow walks in nature. Diets should emphasize fresh, seasonal, lightly cooked vegetables, ideally prepared at home. Meals should be slowly savored along with wholesome conversation. Deep restful sleep should be prioritized, especially in the winter months.

[1] Unschuld, P.U. & Tessenow, H. (2003). *Huang Di Nei Jing Su Wen*. University of California Press: Oakland.

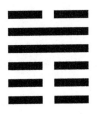

13: What does modern research say about Chinese medicine?

I was the lead researcher on a small Chinese medical study in which two practitioners independently assessed 60 high resolution images of patients' tongues. Our research question was: 'Would two Chinese medicine practitioners looking at the same tongue pictures see the same aspects of the tongues and come to a similar diagnosis?' The answer turned out to be yes. Even though the two practitioners in the study were trained at different Chinese medical universities and had never met in person, their tongue diagnosis ratings showed statistically significant correlations. Studies like this are slowly corroborating aspects of Chinese medicine through scientific research protocols.

One concern about Chinese medicine that is often raised is that it is not evidence-based. This is despite the more than two millennia of historical evidence documenting the safe and effective use of Chinese medicine. This criticism is of course valid if we narrowly define evidence-based medicine to be 'research evidence from meta-analyses and randomized controlled trials'. Chinese medicine is just beginning to accumulate this type of evidence. However, over the last twenty years scientific research into Chinese medicine has begun to flourish, and acupuncture research is growing exponentially. Acupuncture research is even outpacing some biomedical evidence based research.[2]

Most people assume that every routine biomedical intervention is evidence based. However, a recent study found that nearly half of all biomedical interventions are in fact not based on scientific evidence.[1] It would be unwise to refuse these historically safe and effective biomedical interventions simply because they have not been validated by a meta-analysis or a randomized control trial. A similar case can be made for Chinese medicine.

Acupuncture

Acupuncture has enjoyed the most focused research attention of any Chinese medicine modality. The World Health Organization, based on hundreds of studies demonstrating efficacy and an impressive safety profile, recommends acupuncture for dozens of conditions. These conditions range from addressing chemotherapy adverse reactions to alleviating sciatica (see Appendix A for a full list).

The esteemed Cochrane Library provides high quality and unbiased systematic reviews of evidence on health care interventions. It is generally accepted to be among the most carefully prepared and rigorous sources of systematic review. Cochrane's strict protocols have found enough evidence from current research studies to recommend acupuncture for migraines, tension headaches, peripheral joint osteoarthritis, and chronic prostatitis.

Hundreds of research studies have now demonstrated the effectiveness of acupuncture. But by what mechanism does it achieve its wide-ranging effects? Several biochemical signaling pathways have been shown to be involved in the body's response to the insertion of an acupuncture needle. It is now understood that one of the mechanisms of action of acupuncture needles is to directly stimulate the purinergic signaling system.

This system consists of transporters, enzymes, and receptors responsible for the synthesis, release, action, and extracellular inactivation of predominately adenosine triphosphate (ATP), as well as its extracellular breakdown product, adenosine. The purinergic signaling system is used for cell regulation in all tissues and organ systems in the body. All nerve transmission requires ATP, and the body uses purine levels as a primary background signal to determine both healthy function as well as tissue damage. Acupuncture's influence on this system explains at least part of the mechanism for its effects on the entire body.[2,3,4,5,6]

Neuroanatomical research has shown that acupuncture causes a change in the functional connectivity of the brain and a decrease in activity of the limbic structures associated with stress and illness. It has been demonstrated that acupuncture improves the regulation of the hypothalamus-pituitary-adrenal axis, which is the major neuroendocrine system that controls reactions to stress as well as regulating many physiological processes, including digestion, the immune system, mood, emotions, sexuality, energy storage, and energy expenditure. Acupuncture has also been shown to modulate activity of the parasympathetic nervous system, which regulates rest, relaxation, digestion, and tissue healing.[2,7,8,9]

Another recent discovery, by the neurobiologist Dr Qiufu Ma and his team at Harvard medical school, found that a specific type of neuron must be present for an acupuncture needle to trigger an anti-inflammatory response via the vagal-adrenal axis, a signaling pathway in the nervous system.[10] By degrees, researchers are expanding our insight into how an acupuncture needle inserted into a patient's hand, for example, can create a cascade of effects throughout the entire body. To stay up to date on the latest evidence-based acupuncture research, visit the excellent <www.evidencebasedacupuncture.org>.

Herbal medicine

Chinese herbal formulas have had very few double-blind placebo-controlled trials as well as few trials using an adequate research methodology. Because of this, the effectiveness of Chinese herbal medicine, especially herbal substances that have been combined into a formula, remains poorly documented by evidence based medicine.[11]

There have been very few research studies documenting the safety of Chinese herbal medicine. The Cleveland Clinic conducted a seven-year study of every one of their patients taking Chinese herbal medicine. To do this, the clinic monitored every patient's liver and kidney function. During the course of the study, they did not encounter a single lab result showing either liver or kidney dysfunction.[12]

There has been significantly more research into individual herbal substances. Researchers tend to limit themselves to studying single substances because each individual herb routinely contains dozens of bioactive ingredients. Studying an herbal formula - typically 10 to 20 substances each of which comprises dozens of bioactive ingredients, each of which combines with other bioactive ingredients while the mixture is being prepared - results in a bewildering level of complexity for researchers.

Another incentive for studying individual herbs is that they have drawn increasing interest as a source for novel pharmaceuticals. This is unsurprising considering that many modern drugs are derivatives of individual herbal medicines. Below we will examine research into three Chinese herbal substances.

The awarding of the 2015 Nobel Prize to Dr Tu Youyou for the discovery and development of artemisinin, the potent bioactive antimalarial derived from the Chinese herbal substance Qing Hao (Artemisia annuae Herba), was a watershed moment for Chinese herbal medicine research.[13] The use of Qing Hao for addressing malarial conditions was first documented in *Zhou Hou Jiu Zu Fang* (A Handbook of Prescriptions for Emergencies) written by the famous Chinese medical physician Ge Hong in the Eastern Jin Dynasty (317- 420 CE).

Dr Tu even used the original low temperature extraction method recommended in this classical text. She found that switching to an extraction method without the use of heat made her solution 100 per cent effective against malaria in animal models. Antimalarials derived from her work now help combat the estimated 212 million new cases of malaria contracted every year.[14,15,16]

Chinese medicine has been treating symptoms of diabetes since the Han dynasty (206 BCE – 220 CE).[17] Since that time hundreds of formulas have been developed, many of which are still being used effectively today.[18] These formulas often contain the Chinese medicinal Huang Lian (Coptidis Rhizoma). This has been studied extensively and has demonstrated hypoglycemic (blood sugar-lowering) as well as hypolipidemic (cholesterol-lowering) properties.

Berberine, one of the bioactive ingredients in Huang Lian, has been shown to regulate glucose levels so effectively that it is comparable to current first-line diabetic treatments.[19,20] Berberine's effect is likely due to its ability to target glucose metabolism through both insulin-dependent and-independent pathways. It also increases insulin sensitivity, insulin secretion, and glucose uptake. Finally, it can modulate liver metabolic function through the regulation of gene expression, reduce intestinal glucose uptake, and modulate the gut microbiota composition (through antimicrobial activity), among other actions.[13]

Coptisine, another bioactive ingredient in Huang Lian, exerted the potential to be an 'anti-cancer, anti-inflammatory, coronary artery disease ameliorating or anti-bacterial drug through regulating the signaling transduction of (metabolic) pathways'.[21] Berberine and coptisine are just two of Huang Lian's estimated 51 bioactive components.[22] Researchers are currently investigating the remaining components and it is remarkable that these multi-system biological effects are derived from the root of such a simple and easily grown plant.

Cardiovascular disease and cerebrovascular disease are among the leading causes of death in the United States and worldwide. The Chinese herbal medicinal, Dan Shen (Salviae Miltiorrhizae Radix), has historically been utilized in the prevention and treatment of these type of diseases.[23] Dan Shen, whether through oral ingestion or sometimes even as a direct injection, has been the subject of extensive clinical study in China. Positive clinical findings have been reported for ischemic stroke, angina pectoris, intercranial hematoma, and acute myocardial infarction, among others.[25,26,27]

A small herbal formula with the primary ingredient of Dan Shen, along with the Chinese medicinals San Qi (Panax notoginseng) and Bing Pian (Borneolum), was the first herbal formula to be approved for phase II clinical trials by the US Food and Drug Administration.[13,28] This is especially significant because it was not an isolated bioactive component extracted from the 50 estimated bioactive components of Dan Shen that was used in the trial - the entire crude herb (along with the other two medicinals in their intact state) was tested.[29]

This formula's efficacy and lack of side effects propelled it through its clinical trials, and it completed phase III trials in 2016.[23] Phase III trials are the last phase of testing needed before the formula's clinical trial results are submitted to regulatory authorities for approval for use in the general population.

Qi gong and tai ji quan

There has been increasing research interest in the movement-based and embodied contemplative practices of Chinese medicine. Preliminary research suggests that using qi gong may help with depression, anxiety, lung function, and physical function in people with chronic obstructive pulmonary disorder (COPD). A 2020 review of 31 studies (3,045 participants) looked at the effect of adding qi gong to a standard treatment for COPD. The review found that adding qi gong improved lung function, quality of life, and ability to exercise.

A 2020 review examined two small studies to determine if qi gong could have effects on patients with fibromyalgia. The first study (89 participants) found that six months of qi gong practice reduced pain, improved sleep quality, and enhanced physical and mental function. The second study (57 participants) found that seven weeks of practice resulted in decreased pain, decreased anxiety, and improved quality of life.

A 2017 review involving 22 studies (1,751 participants) assessed the impact qi gong practice had on cancer patients. The review found that qi gong was promising for managing physical and psychological symptoms related to cancer and the side effects of its conventional treatment.

A 2020 review of four studies (593 participants) with substance use disorders found that qigong appeared to have a more positive effect on reducing anxiety than medication or no treatment. In addition, the review found that qi gong led to significant improvement in depressive symptoms when compared to no treatment. The research also indicates that qi gong appears to be a very safe activity, even for patients with chronic diseases or elderly patients.[34]

Research suggests that the gentle movements and mental focus cultivated by tai ji quan practitioners have wide ranging health benefits. Studies found with high-certainty evidence that tai ji quan reduces the number of people who experience falls by 20 per cent (based on eight studies involving 2,677 participants). A 2015 review (543 participants) concluded that tai ji quan reduces pain and stiffness in patients with osteoarthritis. Updated 2019 guidelines from the American College of Rheumatology and the Arthritis Foundation now strongly recommend tai ji quan for the management of knee and hip osteoarthritis.

A 2020 review (1,853 participants) evaluated patients who were 60 years or older with cardiovascular disease. The review found that tai ji quan was better than standard care or other types of exercise for improving quality of life and psychological well-being. A 2019 review (656 participants) looked at tai ji quan in the early stages of dementia in older adults. The short-term effect of tai ji quan on the overall cognition of people with mild cognitive impairment was found to be beneficial. Like much of the research into other Chinese medicine modalities, the qi gong and tai ji quan studies tend to be small and invariably the authors of these studies indicate that more research is needed to assess these practices fully.[35]

Cupping, gua sha, and tui na

As we examine modalities such as cupping, gua sha and tui na, research quality and quantity begins to dwindle, in terms of clinical studies as well as investigation into mechanism of action. The most prominent study on cupping was a 2011 review that found cupping therapy significantly reduced low back pain and cancer pain in comparison to painkillers and other standard treatments.[30] Many theories have been suggested to explain the effects of cupping therapy, although researchers have been unable to determine a decisive mechanism.[31]

A small study from 2007 using laser doppler imaging found that gua sha treatment increased local microcirculation. The study proposed that this increase in circulation may play a role in the local and distal decreases in pain experienced by the subjects. Researchers concede that the biomechanism of gua sha is still unidentified, but it may be due - at least in part - to the release of nitric oxide. Nitric oxide is recognized as a potent endogenous vasodilator and plays a role in neurotransmission, platelet aggregation, innate immunity, and inflammation.[32,33]

There have been a few small studies demonstrating the pain-relieving effects of tui na therapy, mostly for low back and neck pain. These small studies were promising enough that a large, randomized, single-blind, parallel-controlled study of tui na for the treatment of chronic low back pain is currently being conducted. This well-designed study, when it is completed, will anchor the research base of tui na therapy.[36]

Other modalities

Unfortunately, there are no significant research studies for moxibustion, Chinese medical nutrition, or the multiple practices comprising yang sheng. With the growing interest in Chinese medicine, it is likely that that these pillars of the medicine will also begin to gather their own research bases over the next few years.

1 Prasad, v, Ioannidis, J.P. (2014). Evidence-based de-implementation for contradicted, unproven, and aspiring healthcare practices, *Implement Sci* 9:1, doi:10.1186/1748-5908-9-1.

2 Koppelman, M. (N.D.). Acupuncture: An Overview of Scientific Evidence, available at <https://www.evidencebasedacupuncture.org/acupuncture-scientific-evidence/> [Accessed 02/12/2023].

3 Wikipedia (N.D.). Purinergic signaling, available at <https://en.wikipedia.org/wiki/Purinergic_signalling> [Accessed 02/12/2023].

4 Verkhratsky, A., Burnstock, G. (2014). Biology of purinergic signalling: Its ancient evolutionary roots, its omnipresence and its multiple functional significance, *Bioessays*, 36:697–705.

5 Sperlagh, B., Csolle, C. et al. (2012). The role of purinergic signaling in depressive disorders, *Neuropsychopharmacologia Hungarica*, 14(4): 231–8.

6 Burnstock, G. (2014). Purinergic signaling in acupuncture, *Science*, 346(6216 Suppl):S23–S25.

7 Cho, Z.H., Hwang, S.C., Wong, E.K. et al. (2006). Neural substrates, experimental evidences and functional hypothesis of acupuncture mechanisms, *Acta Neurol Scand*, 113:370–7.

8 Lund, I., Lundeberg, T. (2016). Mechanisms of *Acupuncture*. *Acupuncture and Related Therapies*, 4(4):26-30.

9 Wikipedia (N.D.). Hypothalamic–pituitary–adrenal axis, available at <https://en.wikipedia.org/wiki/Hypothalamic–pituitary–adrenal_axis> [Accessed 02/12/2023].

10 The neuron is a PROKR2-Cre marked sensory neuron. Liu, S., Wang, Z., Su, Y. et al. (2021). A neuroanatomical basis for electroacupuncture to drive the vagal–adrenal axis, *Nature*, 598, 641–645.

[11] Shang, A.J., Huwiler, K., Nartey, L. et al. (2007). Placebo-controlled trials of Chinese herbal medicine and conventional medicine—comparative study, *International Journal of Epidemiology*, 36(5):1086–1092.

[12] Cleveland Clinic (2021). What you should know about Chinese herbs, available at <https://health.clevelandclinic.org/what-you-should-know-about-chinese-herbs/> [Accessed 02/12/2023].

[13] Wang, J., Wong, Y., Liao, F. (2018). What has traditional Chinese medicine delivered for modern medicine? *Expert Reviews in Molecular Medicine*, 20, E4. doi:10.1017/erm.2018.3.

[14] Collaboration Research Group for Qinghaosu (1982). Chemical studies on Qinghaosu, *Journal of Traditional Chinese Medicine*, 2:3–8.

[15] Tu, Y. (2016). Artemisinin – a gift from traditional Chinese medicine to the world (Nobel Lecture), *Angewandte Chemie*, 55:10210–10226.

[16] Hoshen, M. (2004). Artesunate combinations for malaria, *Lancet*, 363(9410):737.

[17] Tong, X.L., Dong, L., Chen, L. et al. (2012). Treatment of diabetes using traditional Chinese medicine: past, present and future, *American Journal of Chinese Medicine*, 40(5):877–886.

[18] Li, W.L., Zheng, H.C., Bukuru, J. et al. (2004). Natural medicines used in the traditional Chinese medical system for therapy of diabetes mellitus, *Journal of Ethnopharmacology*, 92(1):1–21.

[19] Dong, H., Wang, N., Zhao, L. et al. (2012). Berberine in the treatment of type 2 diabetes mellitus: a systemic review and meta-analysis, *Evidence-Based Complementary and Alternative Medicine*, DOI: 10.1155/2012/591654.

20 Lan, J.R., Zhao, Y.Y., Dong F.X. et al. (2015). Meta-analysis of the effect and safety of berberine in the treatment of type 2 diabetes mellitus, hyperlipemia and hypertension, *Journal of Ethnopharmacology*, 161:69–81.

21 Metabolic pathways such as: NF - κB, MAPK, PI3K/Akt, NLRP3 inflammasome, RANKL/RANK and Beclin 1/Sirt1; see Wu, J., Luo, Y., Deng, D. (2019). Coptisine from Coptis chinensis exerts diverse beneficial properties: A concise review, *J Cell Mol Med*, 23(12):7946-7960.

22 Meng, F.C., Wu, Z.F., Yin, Z.Q. et al. (2018). Coptidis rhizoma and its main bioactive components: recent advances in chemical investigation, quality evaluation and pharmacological activity, *Chin Med*, 13:13, DOI: 10.1186/s13020-018-0171-3.

23 Liu, Y., Yin, H.J., Shi, D.Z. et al. (2012). Chinese herb and formulas for promoting blood circulation and removing blood stasis and antiplatelet therapies, *Evidence-Based Complementary and Alternative Medicine*, DOI: 10.1155/2012/184503.

24 Lei, X., Chen, J., Liu, C.X. et al. (2014). Status and thoughts of Chinese patent medicines seeking approval in the US market, *Chinese Journal of Integrative Medicine*, 20:403–408.

25 Sun, M., Zhang, J.J., Shang, J.Z. et al. (2009). Clinical observation of Danhong injection (herbal TCM product from radix *Salviae miltiorrhizae* and *Flos Carthami tinctorii*) in the treatment of traumatic intracranial hematoma, *Phytomedicine*, 16(8):683–689.

26 Liao, P., Wang, L., Guo, L. et al. (2015). Danhong injection (a Traditional Chinese Patent Medicine) for acute myocardial infarction: a systematic review and meta-analysis, *Evidence-Based Complementary and Alternative Medicine*, DOI: 10.1155/2015/646530.

[27] Wang, H., Ren, S., Liu, C. et al. (2016). An overview of systematic reviews of Danhong injection for ischemic stroke, *Evidence-Based Complementary and Alternative Medicine*, DOI: 10.1155/2016/8949835.

[28] Writing Group of Recommendations of Expert Panel from Chinese Geriatrics Society on the Clinical Use of Compound Danshen Dripping Pills (2017). Recommendations on the clinical use of compound Danshen dripping pills, *Chinese Medical Journal*, 130(8):972–978.

[29] Wang, X.H., Morris-Natschke, S.L., Lee K.H. et al. (2007). New developments in the chemistry and biology of the bioactive constituents of Tanshen, *Medicinal Research Reviews* 27:133–148.

[30] Kim J.I., Lee, M.S., Lee, D.H. et al. (2011). Cupping for Treating Pain: A Systemic Review, *Evidence-Based Complementary and Alternative Medicine*, DOI:10.1093/ecam/nep035.

[31] Al-Bedah, A.M.N., Elsubai, I.S., Qureshi, N.A. et al. (2018). The medical perspective of cupping therapy: Effects and mechanisms of action, *J Tradit Complement Med*, 30;9(2):90-97.

[32] Nielsen, A., Knoblauch, N.T., Dobos, G.J. (2007). The effect of gua sha treatment on the microcirculation of surface tissue: a pilot study in healthy subjects, Explore, 3(5):456-66.

[33] Chu, E.C.P., Wong, A.Y.L., Sim, P. et al. (2021). Exploring scraping therapy: Contemporary views on an ancient healing - A review, *J Family Med Prim Care*, 10(8):2757-2762.

[34] National Center for Complementary and Integrative Health (N.D.). Qigong: What you need to know, available at <www.nccih.nih.gov/health/qigong-what-you-need-to-know> [Accessed 02/18/2023].

[35] National Center for Complementary and Integrative Health (N.D.). Tai Chi: What you need to know, available at <https://www.nccih.nih.gov/health/tai-chi-what-you-need-to-know> [Accessed 02/19/2023].

[36] US National Library of Medicine (2022). A Study on the Effectiveness of Tuina in Managing Chronic Low Back Pain, available at <https://clinicaltrials.gov/ct2/show/NCT05363579> [Accessed 02/19/2023].

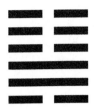

14: Why bother with yang sheng? (Why take care of my 'rental car'?)

My teacher, Dr Angela C. Wu, always reminded her patients that we do not get to keep our bodies forever and that someday soon we will have to return what she called our 'rental cars'. What should we do with our 'rental car'? There are really only three things we can do - we can look after it, use it for worthwhile endeavors, or run it into the ground.

There is nothing in your life that does not involve your body and mind. If the function of the body and mind can be significantly improved then everything worth caring about - relationships, the capacity to work, sleep, have sex, and everything else - gets better. Chinese medicine is replete with methods to improve our mental and physical health. The practices and lifestyle modifications of yang sheng provide a complete framework for 'nurturing life'. Yang sheng practices offer personalized and seasonal guidelines for diet, exercise, sleep, sexual behavior, and more - all aimed at increasing the quantity of our lifespans and quality of our health-spans.

You may use latest research as a guide to help you choose different aspects of Chinese medicine to nurture your health. Perhaps you have recently been diagnosed with cancer. You may take up qi gong practice because of the promising research showing its benefits in managing physical and psychological symptoms related to your cancer. Or if you suffer from debilitating migraines, you may consider seeking acupuncture treatment. Or you may have a family history of cardiovascular disease, so you seek out a Chinese herbalist to see if an herbal formula containing Dan Shen might be appropriate as a preventative measure.

Once you have achieved a modicum of health this is not an endpoint. Health is just potential - a prerequisite for accomplishing worthwhile things in this life. What will you do with that potential? Health affords us the opportunity to engage in fruitful endeavors: building and deepening relationships, parenting, engaging in meaningful work, gathering knowledge, mentoring others, taking care of our fellow humans and non-humans, travelling, appreciating art…with flourishing health the possibilities become endless.

Maintaining your health is not only a preventive measure for disease, but also offers a strong foundation for recovery if you experience a serious disease or injury. A patient in her late 40s who I saw this week has unfortunately not been cultivating her health. She has been squandering it by smoking since her teens, eating fast food, and diligently avoiding exercise. She is 100 pounds (45 kilograms) overweight.

She was recently diagnosed with stage four cervical cancer. Her eldest daughter is eight months pregnant. She wants more than anything to be a healthy first-time grandmother. Regrettably, we cannot beg, borrow, or steal health when we confront a significant illness like cancer. Health must already be cultivated and in place. This patient has a great distance to cover in a short amount of time to reclaim her health, at a time when she needs it more than ever.

It is easy to understand that we should avoid dissipating our health. It is more difficult to know how exactly to cultivate it. Some people need to go on a silent meditation retreat. Other people need to start lifting heavy weights. Some people need to go to bed earlier. Others need to go out to dinner with new friends. Some need to eat dense heavy meals. Others need to eat light clear soups. Some need to go out for a run. Others need to stay at home and read a good book sitting by a warm fire. You may be all these people, just at different times in your life. The challenge is to know what you require at each moment to cultivate health.

Fortunately, we can use the principal theory of Chinese medicine - yin and yang - to identify what behaviors to pursue and when. You may want to navigate this dynamic balance on your own or seek advice and treatment from a practitioner of Chinese medicine. Always remain flexible in your health promoting efforts. Strive to perfectly balance the changing yin-yang patterns as they unceasingly arise and fall throughout your life.

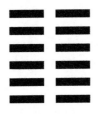

15: How do I find a good Chinese medicine practitioner?

Hopefully you are already working with an exceptional practitioner of Chinese medicine. However, if you are looking for one, the best way to find a skilled practitioner is through your local social network. Let this network know you are seeking a referral and the condition you need help with. Ideally one name will come up over and over from different members of your group. You can do the same for your local social media group.

Word of mouth from your social network is the ideal way to find a practitioner. If that route is not available, another way to find a good practitioner is by going to your local health food store and asking employees for recommendations. People who seek out Chinese medicine tend to be the same type of people that do something extra for their health like shopping at a health food store. Employees of that store hear a lot of talk about health care practitioners and can therefore be invaluable sources of recommendations.

As an aside, one of my translators in China thought it was very strange that in the US we have a gigantic regular grocery store and nearby a small health food store. She wondered 'What is in that huge store?' I was too embarrassed to tell her the answer.

You can also search for a practitioner near you through these directories:

Most of the US: <www.nccaom.org/find-a-practitioner-directory/>
California: <search.dca.ca.gov/advanced>
Canada: <cmaac.ca/public/find-a-practitioner>
Europe: <etcma.org/find-a-member/>
UK: <https://acupuncture.org.uk>
Australia: <www.acupuncture.org.au/find-a-practitioner>
New Zealand: <www.nzasa.org/find-a-practitioner/>

Whichever method you use, consider reaching out and interviewing your potential provider before your appointment. Things to ask:

- Tell me about your background and how you got into this field?
- How long have you been in practice? (Established practitioners are ideal but newer practitioners with strong mentorship ties should also be considered)
- What are the most common conditions you treat?
- Do you have experience treating my condition?
- How many patients do you see in a day?

Perhaps more significant than their answers are how they answer your questions. How comfortable you are with their communication style is important. You are going to trust them with your health, so you should feel comfortable with them as a person. Your ideal practitioner is consistent with their words, compassionate, and humble.

Epilogue

We have completed our tour of the peaks that comprise the Chinese medical landscape. I hope this brief guide provides a foundation for a healthful engagement with the medicine. In the next and final section, you will find recommendations for further reading on any Chinese medicine topic that you would like to explore in more depth. My hope is that whether you are looking to bolster your already good health, or you are seeking relief from a recalcitrant disease, this book will help guide your relationship with this ancient medicine.

Suggestions for further reading:

Overviews of Chinese medicine

The Web That Has No Weaver by Ted Kaptchuck – a good overview of the theories of Chinese medicine

Traditional Chinese Medicine by Paul Unschuld – a good historical overview of Chinese medicine

The Foundations of Chinese Medicine by Giovanni Maciocia – a core Chinese medicine textbook

Between Heaven and Earth by Harriet Beinfield and Efrem Korngold – psychological models of Chinese medicine

History

Chinese Medicine and Healing: An Illustrated History by TJ Hinrichs (Editor), Linda L. Barnes (Editor)

Acupuncture and Chinese Medicine: Roots of Modern Practice by Charles Buck

Neither Donkey nor Horse: Medicine in the Struggle over China's Modernity by Sean Hsiang-lin Lei

Diagnosis

Diagnosis in Chinese Medicine: A Comprehensive Guide by Giovanni Maciocia

Atlas of Chinese Tongue Diagnosis by Barbara Kirschbaum

Chinese Pulse Diagnosis: A Contemporary Approach by Leon Hammer

Fukushin and Kampo: Abdominal Diagnosis in Traditional Japanese and Chinese Medicine by Nigel Dawes

Acupuncture

Acupuncture Points Handbook: A Patient's Guide to the Locations and Functions of over 400 Acupuncture Points by Deborah Bleecker

A Manual of Acupuncture by Peter Deadman, Mazin Al-Khafaji, and Kevin Baker

Pictorial Atlas of Acupuncture: An Illustrated Manual of Acupuncture Points by Yu-Lin Lian, Chun-Yan Chen, Michael Hammes, and Bernhard C. Kolster

Moxibustion

Moxibustion: The Power of Mugwort Fire by Lorraine Wilcox

Moxibustion: A Modern Clinical Handbook by Lorraine Wilcox

Illustrated Moxibustion Therapy: A Natural Way of Prevention and Treatment through Traditional Chinese Medicine by Xuezhong Duan

Herbal medicine

Chinese Herbal Medicine: Materia Medica by Dan Bensky and Andrew Gamble

Chinese Herbal Medicine: Formulas & Strategies by Volker Scheid, Dan Bensky, Andrew Ellis and Randall Barolet

Chinese Medical Herbology & Pharmacology by John K. Chen, Tina T. Chen, Laraine Crampton, Charles Funk, and Rick Friesen

Chinese Herbal Formulas and Applications by John K. Chen, Tina T. Chen, Minh Nguyen, Lily Huang, Jimmy Chang, Rick Friesen, and Chien-Hui Liao

The Way of Chinese Herbs by Michael Tierra

Cupping

A Practical Guide to Cupping Therapy: A Natural Approach to Heal Through Traditional Chinese Medicine by Zhongchao Wu

Traditional Chinese Cupping Therapy by Ilkay Chirali

Gua sha

Gua Sha: A Traditional Technique for Modern Practice by Arya Nielsen

Gua Sha: A Complete Self-treatment Guide by Clive Whitham

Diet

The Asian Diet by Jason Bussell

The Tao of Healthy Eating by Bob Flaws

Chinese Nutrition Therapy by Joerg Kastner

Healing with Whole Foods by Paul Pitchford

Chinese Nutritional Strategies app (Apple and Android) by Toby Daly

Qi gong

The Way of Qigong: The Art and Science of Chinese Energy Healing by Kenneth Cohen

Live Well Live Long by Peter Deadman

Chinese Healing Exercises: A Personalized Practice for Health & Longevity by Steven Cardoza

Tai ji quan

The Harvard Medical School Guide to Tai Chi: 12 Weeks to a Healthy Body, Strong Heart, and Sharp Mind by Peter Wayne and Mark Feurest

The Complete Book of Tai Chi Chuan: A Comprehensive Guide to the Principles and Practice by Wong Kiew Kit

Tui na

Tui Na: A Manual of Chinese Massage Therapy by Sarah Pritchard

Chinese Tui Na Massage: The Essential Guide to Treating Injuries, Improving Health & Balancing Qi by Xiang Cai Xu

Yang sheng

Live Well Live Long by Peter Deadman

Yang Sheng: The Art of Chinese Self-Healing: Ancient Solutions to Modern Problems by Katie Brindle

Appendix A: The World Health Organization on acupuncture

The World Health Organization recommends acupuncture for these diseases, symptoms, or conditions because acupuncture has been 'prove[n] – through controlled trials – to be an effective treatment':

Adverse reactions to radiotherapy and/or chemotherapy

Allergic rhinitis (including hay fever)

Biliary colic

Depression (including depressive neurosis and depression following stroke)

Dysentery, acute bacillary

Dysmenorrhea, primary

Epigastric pain, acute (in peptic ulcer, acute and chronic gastritis)

Facial pain (including craniomandibular disorders)

Headache

Hypertension, essential

Hypotension, primary

Induction of labor

Knee pain

Leukopenia

Low back pain

Malposition of fetus, correction of

Morning sickness

Nausea and vomiting

Neck pain

Pain in dentistry (including dental pain and temporomandibular dysfunction)

Periarthritis of shoulder

Postoperative pain

Renal colic

Rheumatoid arthritis

Sciatica

Sprain

Stroke

Tennis elbow

Diseases, symptoms, or conditions for which the World Health Organization recommends acupuncture because its therapeutic effect has been shown, although further proof is needed:

Abdominal pain (in acute gastroenteritis or due to gastrointestinal spasm)

Acne vulgaris

Alcohol dependence and detoxification

Bell's palsy

Bronchial asthma

Cancer pain

Cardiac neurosis

Cholecystitis, chronic, with acute exacerbation

Cholelithiasis

Competition stress syndrome

Craniocerebral injury, closed

Diabetes mellitus, non-insulin-dependent

Earache

Epidemic hemorrhagic fever

Epistaxis, simple (without generalized or local disease)

Eye pain due to subconjunctival injection

Female infertility

Facial spasm

Female urethral syndrome

Fibromyalgia and fasciitis

Gastrokinetic disturbance

Gouty arthritis

Hepatitis B virus carrier status

Herpes zoster (human (alpha) herpes virus 3)

Hyperlipemia

Hypo-ovarianism

Insomnia

Labor pain

Lactation, deficiency

Male sexual dysfunction, non-organic

Meniere disease

Neuralgia, post-herpetic

Neurodermatitis

Obesity

Opium, cocaine, and heroin dependence

Osteoarthritis

Pain due to endoscopic examination

Pain in thromboangiitis obliterans

Polycystic ovary syndrome (Stein–Leventhal syndrome)

Postextubation in children

Postoperative convalescence

Premenstrual syndrome

Prostatitis, chronic

Pruritus

Radicular and pseudo radicular pain syndrome

Raynaud syndrome, primary

Recurrent lower urinary-tract infection

Reflex sympathetic dystrophy

Retention of urine, traumatic

Schizophrenia

Sialism, drug-induced

Sjogren syndrome

Sore throat (including tonsillitis)
Spine pain, acute
Stiff neck
Temporomandibular joint dysfunction
Tietze syndrome
Tobacco dependence
Tourette syndrome
Ulcerative colitis, chronic
Urolithiasis
Vascular dementia
Whooping cough (pertussis)

Diseases, symptoms, or conditions for which only individual controlled trials report some therapeutic effects; the World Health Organization recommends acupuncture for these when treatment by conventional and other therapies is difficult:

Chloasma
Choroidopathy, central serous
Color blindness
Deafness
Hypophrenia
Irritable colon syndrome
Neuropathic bladder due to spinal cord injury
Pulmonary heart disease, chronic
Small airway obstruction

Bibliography

Bensky, D., Clavey, S., Stoger, E. et al. (2004). *Chinese Herbal Medicine: Materia Medica*. Eastland Press: Seattle.

Chirali, I. (2014). *Traditional Chinese Cupping Therapy*. Churchill Livingstone: Kindle Desk Publishing

Clear, J. (2018). *Atomic Habits: An Easy & Proven Way to Build Good Habits & Break Bad Ones*. Random House: London.

Cui, Y., Gao, B., Liu, L. et al. (2021). AMFormulaS: an intelligent retrieval system for traditional Chinese medicine formulas, *BMC Med Inform Decis Mak*, 21(2):56.

Daly, T. *Chinese Nutritional Strategies*. iOS app.

Deadman, P. (2016). *Live Well Live Long*. Journal of Chinese Medicine Publications: Hove.

Deadman, P. Al-Khafaji, M. (1998). *A Manual of Acupuncture*. Journal of Chinese Medicine Publications: Hove.

Hammer, L. (2001). *Chinese Pulse Diagnosis: A Contemporary Approach*. Eastland Press: Seattle.

Harper, D. (1998). *Early Chinese Medical Manuscripts: The Mawangdui Medical Manuscripts*. Kegan Paul International: New York.

Jiangsu College of New Medicine (2005). *Zhong Yao Ci Dian*. Shang Hai Science and Technology: Shanghai.

Kaptchuck, T. (2000). *The Web That Has No Weaver*. McGraw Hill: New York.

Kim J.I., Lee, M.S., Lee, D.H. et al. (2011). Cupping for Treating Pain: A Systemic *Review, Evidence-Based Complementary and Alternative Medicine*, DOI:10.1093/ecam/nep035.

Lo, V., & Stanley-Baker, M. (2022). *Routledge Handbook of Chinese Medicine*. Routledge: London.

Mitchell, C., Feng, Y., Wiseman N. (1999). *Shang Han Lun: On Cold Damage*. Paradigm Publications: Brookline.

Nielsen, A. & Wieland, S. (2019). Cochrane reviews on acupuncture therapy for pain: A snapshot of the current evidence, *EXPLORE*, 15(6):434-439.

Nielsen, A. (2013). *Gua Sha: A Traditional Technique for Modern Practice*. Churchill Livingstone: Edinburgh.

National Institutes of Health. (1997). Acupuncture, 15(5):1-34.

World Health Organization (1979). Acupuncture, *World Health*.

Ou, H. (2016). *The First Forty Days: The Essential Art of Nourishing the New Mother*. Abrams Books: New York.

Prasad, V., Ioannidis, J.P. (2014). Evidence-based de-implementation for contradicted, unproven, and aspiring healthcare practices, *Implement Sci*, 9:1, DOI:10.1186/1748-5908-9-1.

Pritchard, S, (2015). T*ui Na: A Manual of Chinese Massage Therapy*. Singing Dragon: London.

Scheid, V., Bensky, D., Ellis, A. et al. (2009). Chinese Herbal Medicine: Formulas and Strategies. Eastland Press: Seattle.
Shang, A., Huwiler, K., Nartey, L. et al. (2007). Placebo-controlled trials of Chinese herbal medicine and conventional medicine—comparative study, *International Journal of Epidemiology*, 36(5):1086–1092.

Unschuld, P. (2019). *Traditional Chinese Medicine*. Columbia University Press: New York.

Unschuld, P. & Tessenow, H. (2011). *Huang Di Nei Jing Su Wen*. University of California Press: Berkely.

Wilms, S. (2016). *Shen Nong Bencao Jing*. Happy Goat Productions: Freeland.

Xu, X.C. (2002). *Chinese Tui Na Massage: The Essential Guide to Treating Injuries, Improving Health & Balancing Qi*. YMAA Publication Center: Wolfboro.

Wu, Z.C. (2017). *A Practical Guide to Cupping Therapy: A Natural Approach to Heal Through Traditional Chinese Medicine*. *Shanghai Press*: Shanghai.

Printed in Great Britain
by Amazon